LUPUS-FRIENDLY DIET

Purposeful Diet For Immune Health. Recipes Cookbook On Knowledge To Live Well, Manage, Strive And Reverse Inflammatory Diseases

DR. CHARLSE BLESSING

DISCLAIMER

The information in this book is meant solely for educational reasons. This book's contents are not meant to be used in place of expert medical advice, diagnosis, or treatment. Any decisions you make about your health must be discussed with a licensed healthcare provider.

Every effort has been made by the author to guarantee that the material in this book is correct and current as of the date of publication. Still, since medical knowledge advances rapidly, new studies might be conducted that change our understanding this illness and how best to manage it with food.

This book may contains references to and mentions of various people, things, websites, organizations, and other entities that the author does not support, advocate, or have any association with. There is no implied sponsorship or collaboration; all references and remarks are made only for informational purposes.

In order to address their individual health concerns, readers are advised to independently verify any information contained in this book and to consult with healthcare specialists. Any negative effects arising from the use or implementation of the material in this book, whether direct or indirect, are not the responsibility of the author or the publisher.

The dietary suggestions and counsel provided in this book are broad in scope and might not be appropriate for every individual. Readers are recommended to seek tailored counsel from trained healthcare specialists as individual health problems and demands differ.

The reader accepts the conditions of this disclaimer by reading this book.

FACTS ABOUT THIS BOOK

For those suffering from lupus, a chronic autoimmune disease, the book "Lupus-Friendly Diet" is an invaluable resource. Its importance stems from its thorough examination of the complex interplay between nutrition and lupus symptom treatment. The early chapters offer a sophisticated perspective on lupus, highlighting the critical role that nutrition plays in determining how the illness progresses. The book lays the groundwork for making educated dietary decisions by exploring the unique nutritional requirements of lupus patients.

The identification and absorption of important nutrients necessary for the management of lupus is a crucial topic discussed in the book. Readers are equipped to make dietary choices that help reduce inflammation associated with lupus by the emphasis on anti-inflammatory foods, omega-3 fatty acids, and essential vitamins and minerals.

By helping readers create customized meal plans that are suited to their unique lupus needs, the book goes beyond theoretical understanding. It helps make dietary recommendations more realistically implemented by addressing issues like quantity control and meal time.

The complex relationship between food triggers and lupus is examined in an extremely insightful section. The book helps readers make better food decisions by offering insights into the recognition and control of these triggers. A chapter on recipes suitable for people with lupus adds even more practical value to the book by providing readers with actual examples of meals that are suited to their dietary requirements.

Recognizing the reality of everyday life for people with lupus, the advice on food planning and preparation is equally crucial. To help readers maintain a lupus-friendly diet even while they are in social situations, the book guides dining out, acknowledging the social aspect of eating. Because living with lupus is a complex condition, the book gains depth from the discussion on supplements, lifestyle issues, and holistic methods of lupus therapy.

"Lupus-Friendly Diet" is all things considered, an invaluable tool that gives readers the information and resources they need to take charge of their condition by making informed dietary decisions. The book encourages a holistic approach to lupus management that goes beyond the boundaries of conventional medical interventions by skillfully fusing scientific insights with useful guidance. This allows people with lupus to take control of their health and well-being.

CHAPTER ONE

OVERVIEW
Knowledge About Lupus

Those who are diagnosed with lupus, a complex autoimmune illness, face numerous obstacles. When the body is not protected by the immune system, it attacks healthy tissues and organs. This results in discomfort, inflammation, and damage that can impact multiple systems, such as the blood cells, joints, skin, kidneys, heart, lungs, and brain. For those who have lupus, care is a continuous balancing act because the condition is unpredictable and frequently causes periods of flare-ups and remissions.

It is essential to comprehend lupus if one hopes to find practical solutions for managing its effects on day-to-day living. It necessitates understanding both the unique characteristics of the illness and the range of symptoms and their possible severity. Every individual with lupus has a different experience with the disease because of this. This intricacy emphasizes the value of a holistic management strategy, and nutrition plays a key role in this multidimensional approach.

Diet's Function in Lupus Management

In recent years, there has been a growing amount of emphasis paid to the connection between food and managing lupus. Although there is no known treatment for lupus, food can significantly improve general well-being, reduce inflammation, and ease symptoms. Anti-inflammatory foods can improve the quality of life for people with lupus by lowering inflammation levels in the body.

Walnuts, flaxseeds, and fatty fish are examples of foods high in omega-3 fatty acids that have been demonstrated to have anti-inflammatory properties. Berries, spinach, and kale are examples of fruits and vegetables high in antioxidants that might help fight oxidative stress, a typical lupus symptom. Furthermore, by giving the body the nutrition it needs to control its reactions, a well-balanced diet can enhance immunological function.

Handling the intricacies of food selections becomes crucial to managing lupus. Avoiding specific trigger foods that can aggravate symptoms may help some people find relief. Alternatively, some nutrients may help lessen the negative effects of lupus on the body. The relationship between nutrition and the immune system emphasizes the necessity for individualized treatment plans that are based on the particular experiences of each patient with lupus.

Objective and Range of the Book
This book aims to provide thorough guidance for anyone looking to adopt a lupus-friendly diet,

given the complex interaction that exists between nutrition and lupus. Its goal goes beyond just providing a compilation of recipes; it explores the science underlying food choices and how those choices affect symptoms of lupus. Readers can make educated choices regarding their dietary patterns by researching the most recent findings and comprehending the subtleties of how food interacts with the immune system.

This book's scope includes not just doable meal plans and recipes, but also thoughtful conversations about the emotional and psychological elements of having lupus. Although the book acknowledges that dietary modifications can be difficult, it offers solutions for getting beyond challenges and developing a healthy relationship with food. In the end, the intention is to enable lupus patients to actively participate in their health by enabling them to make decisions based on their specific requirements and preferences.

CHAPTER TWO

FUNDAMENTALS OF FOODS GOOD FOR LUPUS
Needs for Nutrition in Patients with Lupus:

For those who have lupus, a chronic autoimmune illness that can impact many organs and tissues, proper nutrition is essential. To control symptoms, improve general health, and maybe lessen the effects of the condition, it is imperative to address certain dietary requirements. Patients with lupus frequently experience particular difficulties that make careful dietary planning necessary.

Anti-inflammatory foods are a crucial factor to take into account. Incorporating meals high in omega-3 fatty acids, antioxidants, and anti-inflammatory chemicals can be helpful as lupus involves inflammation in the body. Walnuts, flaxseeds, and fatty fish are among the foods high in omega-3s that help lower inflammation. Fruits and vegetables high in antioxidants, such as kale, spinach, and berries, can aid in scavenging free radicals, which are frequently increased in lupus patients.

A diet that is suitable for people with lupus must also include adequate protein. Protein helps maintain muscular growth, aids in tissue regeneration, and boosts immunological function. Individual dietary constraints and preferences can be taken into consideration when including lean protein sources, such as fish, chicken, beans, and tofu. To prevent deficits and assist their body's healing processes, lupus sufferers must closely watch the amount of protein they consume.

Patients with lupus may require special nutrients in addition to careful monitoring of their vitamin and mineral levels. For example, vitamin D is involved in immunological control, and people with lupus frequently have shortages of this vitamin. To help maintain optimal levels, include foods high in vitamin D, such as dairy products with added fortification, or spend time outside in the sun.

A crucial but sometimes disregarded part of controlling lupus symptoms is staying hydrated. Dehydration may be exacerbated by several lupus treatments, and renal problems and weariness are common in lupus patients. Adequate consumption of fluids promotes general well-being and mitigates the adverse effects of drugs.

A Well-Balanced Diet Is Essential

To support general health and manage the complications of the condition, patients with lupus must maintain a balanced diet. A healthy diet gives you the energy, resilience, and nutrients you need to manage your lupus symptoms and any possible drug side effects.

Patients with lupus can better ensure they get a wide range of vital nutrients by following a varied and well-balanced diet.

Vitamins, minerals, carbs, proteins, and lipids are a few of these. A balanced diet helps prevent shortages that could worsen lupus symptoms because each nutrient has a unique function in supporting biological functioning.

In addition, maintaining a healthy weight is important for those with lupus. A balanced diet helps with this. Certain drugs may result in weight gain, while others may make you feel less hungry. To manage energy levels, joint health, and general well-being, people with lupus can benefit from maintaining a healthy weight by eating a balanced diet that includes the proper kinds and amounts of food.

In addition to supporting the immune system, balanced eating is important for lupus patients whose immune systems are hyperactive. A speedier recovery from illness and stronger defense against infections are two benefits of ensuring a proper diet of vitamins and minerals, such as zinc and vitamin C.

A balanced diet can benefit not only physical health but also mental wellness. Appropriate nutrition is important for maintaining mental clarity and stable mood, as some lupus patients may experience sadness or mood fluctuations. People with lupus may benefit from an omega-3 fatty acid-rich diet, as it has been associated with better mental health.

Typical Food Difficulties for People with Lupus:

Individuals with lupus may experience unique dietary needs that call for careful thought and modification. The possible effect of drugs on taste and appetite is one common problem.

People with lupus must concentrate on nutrient-dense foods to make sure they achieve their nutritional requirements even with reduced intake, as some treatments might cause a decrease in appetite.

The existence of dietary allergies and sensitivities in lupus patients presents another frequent difficulty. Food sensitivities can develop in some lupus patients, which can exacerbate symptoms or lead to flare-ups. Finding and avoiding these trigger foods is essential, and collaborating with dietitians or medical professionals can help develop a customized eating plan that takes into account each person's unique dietary needs.

Lupus patients' top priority is controlling inflammation, which can be exacerbated or lessened by food choices. Saturated fats, refined sugars, and processed carbs are known to increase inflammation; on the other hand, a diet abundant in fruits, vegetables, whole grains, and fats that reduce inflammation can help control inflammation levels. For lupus sufferers to maintain general health and manage their symptoms, finding the ideal balance is crucial.

Patients with lupus may find it difficult to stay hydrated, especially if their drugs or the illness is causing kidney problems. Certain lupus treatments may cause excessive urination, which may result in dehydration. Maintaining kidney function and avoiding problems associated with dehydration requires a regular and sufficient intake of fluids.

Furthermore, nutrient absorption may be hampered by the possible effects of lupus on the gastrointestinal tract. It's important to concentrate on nutrient-dense, easily digestible foods because some lupus patients may have digestive problems. Lupus patients' general health and well-being depend on collaborating with medical professionals to manage digestive issues and maximize nutrient absorption.

CHAPTER THREE

ESSENTIAL MINERALS FOR THE TREATMENT OF LUPUS
Anti-Inflammatory Dietary Items for Lupus Treatment:

Chronic inflammation is a common symptom of lupus and is important for the disease's advancement. A diet low in inflammation is essential for the management of lupus symptoms. Consuming foods high in anti-inflammatory compounds can help lower inflammation, ease pain, and improve general health.

Including a diet high in antioxidant-rich fruits and vegetables is a fundamental component of an anti-inflammatory diet. Brightly colored veggies, leafy greens, and berries are rich in chemicals that help fight oxidative stress, which is a prominent cause of inflammation in lupus patients.

Furthermore, the Mediterranean diet's mainstays, such as tomatoes and olive oil, are recognized for their anti-inflammatory qualities.

Another crucial element of a lupus diet that reduces inflammation is whole grains. Foods high in fiber and minerals, such as quinoa, brown rice, and oats, support intestinal health, which is intimately related to the control of inflammation. Conversely, since refined grains and sugars can worsen inflammation, they should be consumed in moderation.

Omega-3 fatty acids, which have strong anti-inflammatory effects, are abundant in fatty fish, like mackerel and salmon. These fatty acids are helpful in the management of lupus because they affect the immune system and reduce inflammation. A lupus-friendly diet can also benefit greatly from including nuts and seeds, especially walnuts and flaxseeds, which are great providers of omega-3s.

In summary, eating an anti-inflammatory diet means putting an emphasis on whole, nutrient-dense foods and limiting your intake of processed and inflammatory foods. By treating the underlying cause of persistent inflammation, this dietary strategy can make a major contribution to the management of lupus symptoms.

Benefits Of Omega-3 Fatty Acids For Patients With Lupus:

The anti-inflammatory and immune-system-modulating qualities of omega-3 fatty acids make them essential for the management of lupus symptoms. Two essential forms of omega-3 fatty acids, eicosapentaenoic acid (EPA) and docosahexaenoic acid (DHA), are abundant in fatty fish, including trout, salmon, and sardines. In lupus patients, these acids help control the inflammatory response, which may lessen the intensity of symptoms.

Another form of omega-3 fatty acid is alpha-linolenic acid (ALA), which can also be found in plant-based sources such as walnuts, chia seeds, and flaxseeds. ALA can be a crucial component of a lupus-friendly diet, especially for individuals with dietary restrictions, even if it is not as powerful as EPA and DHA in terms of its overall anti-inflammatory effect.

Beyond just reducing inflammation, omega-3 fatty acids have many other advantages. They also promote cardiovascular health, which is important for lupus patients because they may have an increased risk of heart problems. Omega-3s offer a comprehensive strategy for controlling cardiovascular problems associated with lupus by regulating blood coagulation, lowering blood pressure, and improving cholesterol levels.

People who have lupus should make sure they get enough omega-3 fatty acids from a variety of plant- and fish-based sources. Although supplements are available, it is normally advised to receive these nutrients from whole foods to maximize effectiveness and absorption.

Vital Vitamins And Minerals For Patients With Lupus:

It can be difficult for lupus patients to maintain appropriate nutritional levels, and certain vitamins and minerals are essential for sustaining general health. Due in part to sun avoidance and the use of sunblock, many lupus patients are susceptible to vitamin D insufficiency, making vitamin D especially important. Sufficient levels of vitamin D are necessary for the immune system to operate properly and for the health of the bones, two important aspects of managing lupus.

Vitamin C, an antioxidant that boosts the immune system and facilitates the creation of collagen, is also important for lupus sufferers to consume in addition to vitamin D. Fruits are good sources of vitamin C and that can be included in a diet for people with lupus include oranges, strawberries, and kiwis.

For lupus patients, calcium is especially important since they may be more susceptible to osteoporosis as a result of using certain drugs and engaging in less physical activity. Good sources of calcium that should be included in the diet to support bone health are dairy products, fortified plant-based milk, and leafy green vegetables.

Patients with lupus may benefit from taking the minerals magnesium and zinc, which are involved in several physiological processes. Rich dietary sources of these minerals include legumes, nuts, seeds, and whole grains.

For lupus patients to address any deficiencies and promote their general health and well-being, they must maintain a well-balanced diet that includes a variety of nutrient-dense foods. To customize dietary recommendations to meet individual needs, it is advised to interact with dietitians or other healthcare specialists regularly.

CHAPTER FOUR

CREATING A MEAL PLAN FOR PEOPLE WITH LUPUS
Making A Plate That Is Balanced For A Diet-Friendly To Lupus:

Building a balanced plate that meets the specific dietary requirements of people with lupus is the first step in developing a lupus-friendly meal plan. To supply vital vitamins and minerals that support general health, the emphasis should be on combining a range of nutrient-dense foods.

The main components of every meal should include fruits, vegetables, lean meats, and whole grains. These ingredients contain antioxidant and anti-inflammatory qualities, which can be very helpful in controlling lupus symptoms, in addition to being part of a balanced diet.

It is important to consider the ratio of macronutrients (carbohydrates, proteins, and fats) while creating a plate that is suitable for people with lupus. Lean proteins like fish or poultry can supply important amino acids, and whole grains like brown rice or quinoa can be a nutritious source of carbohydrates. Nuts, olive oil, avocados, and other healthy fats can all improve the nutritional value of a dish. Maintaining a balance between these components reduces blood sugar spikes and offers a steady supply of energy, which helps avoid the lupus-related weariness that is frequently experienced.

Furthermore, it is recommended to minimize processed meals, refined carbohydrates, and excessive salt intake in lupus patients due to the possibility of sensitivity to specific foods. This enhances general health and aids in the management of inflammation. To make sure that the balanced plate fits with each person's dietary requirements and lupus symptoms, speaking with a nutritionist or other healthcare professional can offer tailored advice.

Lupus And Portion Control:

Controlling portion sizes is essential for both lupus symptom management and general well-being. Keeping a healthy weight is crucial to reducing stress on the joints, heart, and other affected areas of the body because lupus can impact multiple organs and bodily systems. By limiting portion sizes, one can better control caloric intake and avoid needless weight gain that can worsen symptoms and lower quality of life.

People who have lupus should watch their portion sizes to prevent overindulging, especially when it comes to high-energy meals. The body may get the nutrients it needs without consuming too many calories when a range of nutrient-dense foods are consumed in moderation. For instance, including lean proteins in sensible amounts—like fish or tofu—can supply necessary amino acids without adding to an excessive caloric intake.

Portion management can also aid in improved digestion, which is crucial for lupus patients who may have gastrointestinal problems. Throughout the day, eating smaller, more frequent meals might help control symptoms like discomfort and bloating.

This method also aids in blood sugar stabilization, which lessens the chance of energy slumps and exhaustion—a typical worry for lupus sufferers.

Speaking with a medical expert or registered dietitian can offer individualized advice on portion control that takes into consideration a person's activity level, health status, and nutritional requirements.

This guarantees that the meal plan for people with lupus is customized to meet the specific needs of every person, fostering optimum health and symptom control.

When and How Often to Eat for Lupus:

An effective lupus diet depends on the timing and frequency of meals, which affects energy levels, symptom management, and general well-being. Setting up a regular meal plan can help control blood sugar levels and offer a steady supply of energy throughout the day because lupus symptoms are erratic.

It can be helpful for lupus patients to distribute their meals equally throughout the day at smaller, more regular intervals. This strategy helps avoid energy crashes and weariness, which are frequent problems for lupus patients. Smaller meals are often easier for the body to process and lower the risk of gastrointestinal discomfort, thus it also promotes better digestion.

Meal timing is something that should be carefully considered. A healthy snack in between meals can help control blood sugar levels, while a well-balanced breakfast can speed up metabolism and give you long-lasting energy. If you eat dinner earlier in the evening, it might help you sleep better. This is especially important for those with lupus who may already struggle with sleep difficulties.Additionally, the efficiency of lupus medicine can be affected by meal scheduling considerations. Meal timing should be adjusted to accommodate medication regimens, since certain drugs may need food in the stomach for maximum absorption.

In summary, a key element of a diet suitable for people with lupus is scheduling meals at regular intervals. This method improves general health and well-being in addition to boosting energy levels and managing symptoms. Speaking with a qualified dietitian or other healthcare professional can offer tailored advice, ensuring that meal timing complements individual requirements and maximizes the efficacy of lupus treatment techniques.

CHAPTER FIVE

LUPUS AND FOOD TRIGGERS
How to Recognize and Handle Food Triggers in a Lupus-Friendly Diet

For those with lupus who want to reduce symptoms and enhance their general health, recognizing and controlling dietary triggers is essential. In lupus, an autoimmune illness, healthy tissues are mistakenly attacked by the immune system, resulting in inflammation and a variety of symptoms. A key component of managing lupus is diet since certain foods can worsen inflammation and cause flare-ups.

Recognizing that individual lupus reactions can differ is essential to comprehending the impact of dietary triggers. Although there isn't a single solution that works for everyone, processed meals, high sugar, and certain additives are frequently to blame for lupus flare-ups.

Studies indicate that consuming a diet high in anti-inflammatory foods, like fruits, vegetables, and omega-3 fatty acids, may aid in the management of symptoms. However, diets heavy in refined carbohydrates and saturated fats may exacerbate lupus symptoms by causing inflammation.

Furthermore, lupus sufferers frequently struggle to differentiate between allergies and sensitivities. Whereas sensitivities may cause more subdued reactions, allergies entail an immunological response to a particular protein. Recognizing these two kinds of responses is essential for lupus sufferers. While sensitivities can result in delayed reactions that make it difficult to identify the trigger, allergies can induce instant and severe symptoms. Working with healthcare providers, such as dietitians and allergists, can help with thorough testing to pinpoint particular food triggers and customize a diet for those with lupus.

A Diet Friendly for People with Lupus: Allergies vs. Sensitivities

When it comes to creating a lupus-friendly diet that works for you, it's critical to know the difference between allergies and sensitivities.

Allergies are caused by an overreaction of the immune system to a specific protein, which frequently produces sudden and severe symptoms. Conversely, sensitivities can be more difficult to recognize since they often present as delayed and covert reactions. Due to the potential for both kinds of reactions to exacerbate lupus flares, food decisions must be carefully considered.

Lupus patients experiencing allergic responses may include skin rashes, edema, or more severe symptoms such as dyspnea. To avoid severe responses and adjust the lupus-friendly diet appropriately, allergens must be identified through specialized testing.

Less obvious symptoms of sensitivities include gastrointestinal distress, musculoskeletal pain, and exhaustion. Maintaining an extensive food journal will help identify the relationship between particular foods and these delayed reactions, which will make it easier to remove potential triggers from the lupus-friendly diet.

To identify the type of adverse reaction they are experiencing, people with lupus must work closely with healthcare providers. Food diaries, allergy testing, and elimination diets are helpful resources during this phase. This customized method guarantees that the lupus-friendly diet takes sensitivities into account in addition to allergen avoidance, resulting in a thorough plan for handling food triggers.

Maintaining a Food Journal for an All-Lupus Diet

An essential part of controlling lupus and figuring out the nuances of a lupus-friendly diet is maintaining an exacting food journal. With the help of this application, people can keep a useful and insightful record of their daily food intake, symptoms, and possible causes. Keeping a thorough journal helps people make educated food decisions by highlighting trends and connections between particular meals and lupus flare-ups.

Along with the kinds of food eaten, a thorough food journal should contain information about portion sizes, cooking techniques, and any concomitant symptoms. This information aids in identifying possible offenders who may be aggravating lupus symptoms. It also helps to understand the temporal association between food consumption and symptom exacerbation when meal time and symptom start are recorded.

Since these reactions might not be immediately apparent, a food diary is very helpful in identifying sensitivities. People might identify modest triggers that may contribute to flare-ups of their lupus by keeping a long-term record of their daily eating choices and associated symptoms. Working with medical providers to create a customized lupus-friendly diet and order specific tests is made possible by this knowledge.

To sum up, maintaining a dietary journal allows people with lupus to actively participate in their health care. In the end, it is a useful tool for figuring out patterns, differentiating between allergies and sensitivities, and creating a diet that is lupus-friendly, reduces triggers, and enhances general well-being.

CHAPTER SIX

REMEDY SUITABILITY FOR LUPUS
A Boost Your Day with a Nutrient-Packed Smoothie:

A lupus-friendly breakfast is critical for supplying vital nutrients and long-lasting energy. Have a nutrient-rich smoothie to start your day. Blend spinach or kale, which are high in anti-inflammatory and antioxidant qualities, with a banana to create a natural sweetener.

For more protein and probiotics, mix in a scoop of Greek yogurt and a handful of berries for extra antioxidants. Addition of flaxseeds or chia seeds for omega-3 fatty acids can improve the nutritional profile and aid in the management of lupus-related inflammation.

Quinoa Breakfast Bowl with Fresh Fruits:

A lupus-friendly breakfast can benefit greatly from the addition of quinoa, a versatile and nutrient-dense grain. Make a breakfast bowl with cooked quinoa and a variety of fresh fruits, like sliced bananas, kiwis, and berries, on top. The fruits supply vital vitamins and antioxidants, and the quinoa is a full protein source. For sweetness, you may drizzle with some honey. You could also add some chopped nuts for texture and good fats.

Egg and Vegetable Omelet:

Vegetable omelets are a great way to combine eggs, which are a great source of protein, into a breakfast that is suitable for those with lupus. In a pan with colorful vegetables like bell peppers, tomatoes, and spinach, whisk together the eggs and throw them in.

Vegetables provide vitamins and minerals in addition to flavor. Use olive oil when cooking since it is high in monounsaturated fats, which are good for the heart. You'll have plenty of energy throughout the morning thanks to this omelet's high protein and nutritional content.

Salmon is high in omega-3 fatty acids, which have anti-inflammatory qualities that are advantageous for people with lupus. Try it grilled with quinoa and steamed veggies. A hearty and tasty dinner is made with grilled salmon, quinoa, and a mixture of steamed veggies like broccoli, carrots, and zucchini. The vegetables contribute a range of vitamins and minerals, and the quinoa serves as a full protein source. In addition to being delicious, this well-balanced dish promotes lupus control and general wellness.

Vegetarian Stir-Fry with Tofu:

A vibrant vegetarian stir-fry with tofu is a lupus-friendly lunch or dinner choice. Bell peppers, snap peas, and mushrooms are just a few of the colorful veggies that go well with tofu, a great plant-based protein source. For flavoring, use tamari or low-sodium soy sauce. Add garlic and ginger for their anti-inflammatory qualities. For an added boost of nutrition and fiber, serve the stir-fry over brown rice or cauliflower rice.

Curry with Chicken and Vegetables with Turmeric:

Adding turmeric to meals that are suitable for people with lupus can be beneficial because of its anti-inflammatory qualities. Use turmeric, one of the major spices, to make a curry with chicken and vegetables.

To achieve a flavorful and fulfilling combination, incorporate lean chicken, a variety of vibrant vegetables, and coconut milk. For a full and nutritious supper that promotes inflammatory control, serve the curry over basmati rice or quinoa.

Appetizers and Sweets:

Greek Yogurt Parfait with Berries and Nuts: A wonderful and reviving snack or dessert for those with lupus is a Greek yogurt parfait. Strawberries, blueberries, and raspberries are a few of the berries that you can layer over Greek yogurt. For crunch and healthful fats, add in some almonds or walnuts.

Greek yogurt has probiotics that can help with digestive health in addition to being a healthy source of protein.

Fruit Salad with Mint and Honey Drizzle:

As a zesty and sweet dessert that is suitable for people with lupus, prepare a colorful fruit salad. Mix a variety of fruits, such as mango, pineapple, and watermelon.

For an explosion of flavor, add fresh mint leaves, and sprinkle with honey for sweetness. This dessert offers a variety of vitamins, minerals, and antioxidants from the various fruits in addition to being aesthetically pleasing.

Almond Milk Chia Seed Pudding:

Packed in omega-3 fatty acids, chia seeds form a filling and nutritious pudding. Stir in the chia seeds and almond milk, then refrigerate until the mixture thickens. Add more sweetness and nutrients to the pudding by topping it with sliced fruit or fresh berries. This tasty dessert or snack is suitable for people with lupus and is high in nutrients that promote general health.

CHAPTER SEVEN

MEAL PREPARATION AND PLANNING
Batch Cooking for Convenience:

For those on a lupus-friendly diet, batch cooking is a useful and efficient method. It is cooking big batches of food at once and putting it in the fridge to eat later. Because it cuts down on the amount of time and effort spent in the kitchen each day, this strategy is especially helpful for those who have lupus because it lessens physical stress and exhaustion.

For lupus patients, batch cooking offers several benefits, including the capacity to manage ingredient quality and guarantee adherence to dietary guidelines. When meals are prepared ahead of time, people can select fresh, organic, and lupus-friendly ingredients with care, avoiding preservatives or additives that could aggravate symptoms.

This promotes general health and aids in the efficient management of symptoms associated with lupus.

Furthermore, batch cooking makes portion control possible, which is essential for a diet that is lupus-friendly. Sustaining uniform serving sizes can help with weight control, which is crucial for lupus sufferers because being overweight can aggravate joint pain and exhaustion. Furthermore, eating meals in moderation aids in controlling caloric intake, which is essential for people managing lupus symptoms and any drug side effects.

Batch cooking offers a wide variety of lupus-friendly dishes that may be switched up every week to avoid boredom and provide a well-balanced diet. For those with lupus, who frequently worry about nutrient deficits, this diversity is crucial for ensuring that their needs are met. Patients with lupus can be guaranteed to get a wide range of vitamins and minerals by including whole grains, lean proteins, and a vibrant assortment of fruits and vegetables in their diet.

In conclusion, batch cooking is a useful and effective tactic for lupus sufferers trying to keep up a diet that is compatible with their condition. It gives people the tools they need to take charge of their diet, lowers everyday stress, encourages portion control, and provides a range of nutrient-dense meals that improve general well-being.

Ideas for Lupus Patients Planning Meals:

For those with lupus, meal planning is an invaluable tool that offers an organized way to keep a diet appropriate for their illness while coping with its problems. A few essential strategies can be used to improve efficiency and diet compliance while meal planning for lupus.

To start, it's critical to organize meals so that anti-inflammatory foods are the main course. Certain foods can either worsen or lessen the symptoms of inflammation, which is a hallmark of the autoimmune disease lupus. Including omega-3 fatty acids from walnuts, flaxseeds, and fatty fish can help control inflammation. Including a range of vibrant fruits and vegetables with strong antioxidant content also boosts immunity generally and lowers inflammation.

A key strategy for meal planning with lupus that works well is to emphasize nutrient density. Meal planning offers a chance to optimize nutritional intake because lupus patients may have trouble absorbing specific nutrients. Including foods high in nutrients, such as leafy greens, lean proteins, and whole grains, guarantees that every meal meets certain nutritional demands and promotes general health.

A vital component of managing lupus is staying hydrated, thus using foods high in water content in meal preparations might be advantageous. Foods high in water content, such as celery, cucumbers, and watermelon, not only help you stay hydrated but also give your meals a fresh, interesting taste.

Picking straightforward and simple-to-make meal prep recipes is advised in light of lupus-related exhaustion and energy levels. This allows the person to still enjoy tasty and nutritious meals while putting less physical burden on them. Further streamlining the cooking process can be achieved by using kitchen appliances like quick pots and slow cookers.

To sum up, meal planning for someone with lupus necessitates careful thought and attention to certain dietary requirements. People with lupus can maintain a varied and nourishing diet while managing their illness with ease if they prioritize anti-inflammatory foods, vitamin density, hydration, and ease of preparation.

Making Weekly Meal Schedules:

A vital component of maintaining a diet suitable for people with lupus is planning weekly meals. These plans help people navigate the intricacies of dietary limitations related to lupus structure and direction. A thoughtful meal plan helps people maintain a balanced and pleasurable diet by promoting diversity and ensuring appropriate nourishment.

Including a variety of nutrient-dense meals in a weekly meal plan is crucial for people with lupus. Due to their potential difficulties absorbing certain vitamins and minerals, lupus patients have unique nutritional demands that are met in part by this diversity. A variety of lean proteins, entire grains, fruits, and vegetables guarantee a wide range of vital elements.

Meal plans must emphasize items that reduce inflammation for those who have lupus. Some foods, such as leafy greens, berries, and fatty fish, have anti-inflammatory qualities that can help control inflammation associated with lupus. Incorporating these nutrients into the weekly diet plan enhances general health and strengthens the immune system.

Portion management is also essential for controlling the symptoms of lupus and possible drug side effects. Making a weekly food plan enables people to carefully evaluate portion sizes, which helps them maintain a healthy weight and lessens joint stress. Additionally, it encourages steady calorie consumption, which is crucial for managing lupus.

Another essential element of a successful weekly meal plan for lupus is flexibility. Because lupus symptoms are unpredictable, it's critical to prepare ahead of time and keep simple foods on hand for days when energy levels are low. This flexibility guarantees that people can follow their food plan even when they are experiencing more weariness or discomfort.

In conclusion, careful consideration of nutrient diversity, anti-inflammatory foods, portion management, and flexibility are necessary when designing a weekly meal plan for a lupus-friendly diet. People with lupus can effectively manage their illness and enjoy a varied and nutritious diet by including these components in their planning.

CHAPTER EIGHT

HAVING LUPUS AND DINING OUT
Using Restaurant Menu Navigation:

When dining out, one of the biggest obstacles for people with lupus is figuring out which items on restaurant menus are suitable for their condition. A lot of menus might be confusing, with lots of enticing options that could be detrimental to lupus sufferers. People need to be proactive in learning about menu items and their possible effects on their health to make educated judgments.

Choosing simpler recipes made with whole, unadulterated foods is usually a good choice. When combined with a range of vegetables, grilled proteins like fish or chicken can make for a wholesome and lupus-friendly meal. It is important to be cautious when it comes to seasonings, sauces, and secret components as they may contain compounds that aggravate lupus symptoms. People with lupus can make better decisions about their nutrition by being proactive and asking questions of wait staff.

<u>Expressing Dietary Requirements:</u>

For people with lupus, it's critical to properly communicate dietary requirements when dining out. Many people with lupus are subject to certain dietary restrictions, which may include abstaining from certain foods, preservatives, or additives. It is essential to communicate these restrictions to restaurant workers to make sure that meals are served in a way that is compatible with the customer's lupus-friendly diet. The kitchen staff should also be included in this communication, which should stress the need to prevent cross-contamination and make sure that all cooking surfaces and equipment are safe for people with lupus. A collaborative environment between the patron and the restaurant staff can be fostered by being upfront and honest about dietary preferences. This can help people understand lupus and how it affects food choices. In addition to guaranteeing a safer dining experience, this communication helps the hospitality sector become more aware of lupus.

Making Lupus-Friendly Decisions and Socializing:

It might be difficult to maintain a lupus-friendly diet when interacting with others, particularly at social events or get-togethers held in restaurants. But people with lupus must put their health first while still having fun in social situations. When presented with a variety of choices, choosing meals high in anti-inflammatory components can be a lupus-friendly decision. This might include foods high in omega-3 fatty acids, such as salmon or chia seeds, which can help reduce lupus-related inflammation. Furthermore, going for lighter options—like salads made with an assortment of vibrant vegetables—can still deliver vital nutrients without sacrificing flavor. Maintaining a lupus-friendly diet while socializing with friends and family means striking a balance between living in the moment and making health-conscious decisions. People with lupus can achieve this delicate balance and maintain meaningful social connections without sacrificing their well-being by being proactive in choosing lupus-friendly options and communicating dietary needs during social events.

CHAPTER NINE

HERBAL REMEDIES FOR PATIENTS WITH LUPUS
Supplements Suggested for Patients with Lupus on a "LUPUS-FRIENDLY DIET"

As a chronic autoimmune disease, lupus necessitates a multimodal approach to treatment, including proper supplementation and dietary modifications. The goal of this "LUPUS-FRIENDLY DIET" is to improve general health and reduce symptoms. Several supplements may be extremely important for maintaining the health of lupus sufferers.

Omega-3 fatty acids, which are frequently present in fish oil, are a crucial complement for lupus sufferers. Due to their anti-inflammatory qualities, these fatty acids may be able to lessen the long-term inflammation linked to lupus. According to studies, eating more Omega-3-rich foods may lessen the frequency and intensity of lupus flare-ups. To determine the proper dosage, though, it is imperative to speak with a healthcare professional because taking too much of it could have negative effects.

Another essential supplement for people with lupus is vitamin D. Low vitamin D levels are common in lupus patients, despite the vitamin's critical function in immune system control. Vitamin D deficiency raises the risk of osteoporosis and aggravates lupus symptoms. Under the supervision of a medical practitioner, taking supplements can help sustain ideal levels of Vitamin D, which can improve bone health and possibly lessen the intensity of lupus symptoms.

Probiotics, helpful microorganisms that improve gut health, are also suggested for persons with lupus. An imbalance in the gut microbiota can lead to autoimmune diseases like lupus.

The gut microbiome is critical for immune system function. Probiotic supplements may lessen inflammation and enhance immune system performance by assisting in the restoration of a balanced population of gut bacteria.

Patients with lupus may benefit from taking a high-quality multivitamin in addition to specific nutrients. Lupus and its therapies can often lead to dietary shortages, making a well-rounded multivitamin crucial for covering potential gaps in the diet. To customize the supplement regimen to each person's needs, it is necessary to speak with healthcare professionals because taking too much of some vitamins and minerals might have negative consequences.

Talking with Medical Professionals

Before introducing any supplements into a lupus management strategy, patients need to consult with their healthcare practitioners. Lupus is a complex disorder, and individual responses to supplements can differ. To identify the most appropriate supplementation regimen, healthcare experts can evaluate the patient's unique lupus symptoms, drugs currently being used, and overall health.

Additionally, medical professionals can keep an eye out for any possible conflicts between prescription drugs and supplements. For instance, several supplements may interfere with the efficiency of immunosuppressive drugs typically provided for lupus. It is imperative to have regular check-ups and to be in open conversation with medical specialists to make sure that the supplements selected do not compromise health while complementing the overall treatment plan.

Moreover, medical professionals can carry out the required testing to find any current dietary deficits. This enables a tailored and focused approach to supplements, meeting individual needs and preventing needless overabundance that could be harmful. It's critical to schedule routine check-ins with medical professionals to modify supplement dosages in response to modifications in the patient's condition.

Potential Risks and Benefits

For some with lupus, supplements may be beneficial, but there are hazards to be mindful of as well. Not every supplement is appropriate for every person, and some can worsen specific lupus symptoms or interfere with prescription drugs. For instance, consuming too much vitamin D can be harmful and result in nausea, weakness, and other negative symptoms. Finding the right balance between getting the nutrients you need and staying away from dangerous excesses is crucial.

Conversely, the advantages of well-selected supplements, when used in a "LUPUS-FRIENDLY DIET," can be significant. Among the possible benefits are enhanced immunity, decreased inflammation, and support for general health. When prescribed effectively, omega-3 fatty acids, vitamin D, and probiotics can help create a more all-encompassing and successful lupus care plan.

In the end, deciding whether to include supplements in a lupus treatment plan should be decided after consulting medical professionals. It is important to carefully balance the potential hazards and advantages while taking the patient's particular medical history and health conditions into account. To improve their quality of life and manage their illness more effectively, lupus patients can optimize their dietary and supplement regimen by making educated decisions and working together with healthcare providers frequently.

CHAPTER TEN

LUPUS AND LIFESTYLE FACTORS
Lupus And Exercise:

An important part of treating lupus symptoms and enhancing general health for those who have this autoimmune disease is exercise. While exercising may seem contradictory when managing a chronic condition, modest exercise has been demonstrated to have several advantages for individuals with lupus. Frequent exercise supports cardiovascular health, muscular strength, and joint flexibility—all essential for managing lupus.

For those with lupus, low-impact activities like swimming, strolling, or light yoga can be especially helpful since they lessen the chance of joint injury and physical strain. Engaging in these activities can help with weight management and circulation, two vital aspects of general health. Exercise also encourages the body's natural mood enhancers, endorphins, to be released, which helps counteract depressive and anxious feelings that are frequently connected to long-term conditions like lupus.

But before beginning any new plan, people with lupus must customize their fitness schedule to meet their unique needs and speak with medical professionals. Personalized advice makes sure that the activities selected are appropriate for the person's ability and health situation, as overexertion can worsen symptoms. Exercise can improve both physical and mental well-being when included in a lupus-friendly lifestyle with the appropriate technique.

Techniques for Stress Management:

A lupus-friendly lifestyle must include stress management since stress has been related to an aggravation of lupus symptoms and flare-ups. Prolonged stress can have a deleterious effect on the immune system, which may lead to autoimmune reactions in lupus sufferers. Thus, using efficient stress-reduction strategies is essential for controlling the illness and advancing general health.

Patients with lupus can benefit from mindfulness techniques like deep breathing exercises and meditation to reduce stress. These methods encourage relaxation and can give people a stronger sense of mastery over their feelings and ideas. Stress alleviation can also be facilitated by partaking in enjoyable and calming hobbies like reading, listening to music, or spending time in nature.

It's critical to identify unique stressors and triggers and create a customized stress management strategy. This could entail prioritizing work, creating reasonable goals, and developing the ability to say no when it's necessary.

Getting help from friends, family, or support groups can also be very important for stress management.

People with lupus can build resilience and manage the difficulties brought on by their illness by adopting these coping mechanisms into their everyday lives.

Sufficient Sleep for People with Lupus:

While getting enough good sleep is important for everyone, those with lupus need to pay extra attention to this. The body needs sleep to maintain overall health, control immunological response, and repair and renew cells. Making excellent sleep hygiene a priority is an important lifestyle component for lupus patients, who frequently experience exhaustion and heightened pain sensitivity.

A regular sleep schedule that includes a set bedtime and wake-up time might help your body's internal clockwork more smoothly and enhance the quality of your sleep.

It's crucial to provide a peaceful, quiet sleeping environment free from distractions, bright lights, or loud noises for those with lupus.

Moreover, encouraging better sleep depends on controlling the pain and discomfort brought on by lupus symptoms.

This could entail collaborating with medical specialists to identify the best pain-management techniques, like prescription drugs or physical therapy.

A more peaceful sleep can also be achieved by avoiding stimulants like caffeine close to bedtime and using relaxation techniques like moderate stretching or meditation.

For people with lupus, it is critical to understand how sleep, stress, and general health are all related. Not only does getting enough sleep aid with fatigue management, but it also strengthens the body's resistance to the hardships of having a long-term autoimmune disease. People with lupus can improve their overall quality of life by making sleep a priority as part of their self-care routine.

CHAPTER ELEVEN

TRACKING AND MODIFYING YOUR NUTRITION
Frequent Check-ins with Medical Professionals:

For those who adopt a lupus-friendly diet, routine check-ins with healthcare specialists are essential. Food changes may have varying effects on individuals with lupus, a complex autoimmune illness that can affect the body's organs and systems. Rheumatologists and nutritionists are among the medical professionals who are essential in keeping an eye on the general health of lupus patients.

Healthcare professionals can evaluate the patient's general health, lupus symptoms, and possible advantages or side effects of the lupus-friendly diet during these check-ins. To track kidney function, inflammatory levels, and other markers that are influenced by diet, they might order pertinent blood tests. This continuous assessment aids in customizing food suggestions to each person's unique needs and health state.

Healthcare professionals can also offer advice on how to take drugs in addition to making dietary adjustments. Medication for lupus may interact with certain foods or supplements, reducing their effectiveness or perhaps producing negative side effects. Maintaining regular contact with medical professionals guarantees a complete management strategy for lupus that takes nutritional and medical factors into account.

Monitoring Symptoms and Dietary Adjustments:

Those following a lupus-friendly diet should be diligent in monitoring their symptoms and dietary modifications. Individuals with lupus may experience very different symptoms, and dietary triggers or benefits may not always be immediately apparent.

It is possible to analyze the association between dietary choices and lupus symptoms more accurately by keeping a thorough log of symptoms, daily food intake, and any dietary changes.

People can record the frequency and severity of joint pain, exhaustion, skin rashes, and other lupus-related symptoms during the symptom monitoring process. When modifying the lupus-friendly diet, healthcare professionals can use this knowledge as a helpful source of insight. Dietary recommendations can be adjusted to better meet the needs of the individual by observing patterns in the escalation or alleviation of symptoms.

Furthermore, keeping track of dietary modifications entails recording the particular meals eaten, the amounts ingested, and the supplements used. This thorough documentation helps find helpful foods or detect possible triggers.

People with lupus may find over time that particular foods correlate with changes in symptoms, which can help them decide what to add and what to leave out of their diet.

Changing Your Diet to Fit Your Specific Needs:

The lupus-friendly diet can be dynamically and individually adjusted to suit each person's demands. No two people with lupus are the same, and different dietary needs are influenced by variables like age, gender, general health, and particular lupus symptoms. As such, there is no one-size-fits-all method when it comes to diet-related lupus management.

Customized modifications could include changing the kinds of foods eaten, adjusting portion sizes, or adding particular nutrients that promote general health. For instance, a person with kidney problems associated with lupus might need to pay more attention to how much protein and sodium they eat.

A lupus-friendly diet that is flexible enables people to adjust to changes in their health or changing symptoms.

Healthcare professionals and dietitians with expertise in autoimmune diseases can provide tailored advice based on the patient's past medical records and present state of health. Maintaining regular contact with these specialists guarantees that dietary modifications support overall lupus care and are in line with the person's changing demands. To maximize the benefits of a lupus-friendly diet, continued cooperation with healthcare experts is essential since symptoms and medical conditions might vary over time.

CHAPTER TWELVE

COMPREHENSIVE METHODS FOR HANDLING LUPUS: GOING BEYOND DIET

Combining Complementary Medicines:

Complementary therapies are an essential component of a comprehensive strategy in the field of lupus therapy. While traditional medical care is still important, complementary therapies add to a whole plan that takes care of many aspects of health. These treatments cover a broad spectrum of techniques, such as massage, acupuncture, and herbal supplements, among others.

With roots in traditional Chinese medicine, acupuncture is thought to encourage balance and energy flow inside the body. Conversely, massage therapy can mitigate some of the discomfort related to lupus by promoting relaxation and lowering muscle tension.

Supplements containing herbs, when used sensibly and under medical professionals' supervision, could provide extra help. Some herbs may help control lupus symptoms because of their antioxidant and anti-inflammatory qualities. Combining these complementary therapies with a diet that is suited for people with lupus highlights the need to take a multifaceted approach to overall health. To make sure these behaviors are in line with their entire treatment plan, people must speak with their healthcare team before implementing them.

Mind-Body Link:

Comprehending the complex relationship between the mind and body is fundamental to integrative methods of managing lupus. The fact that stress is a known cause of lupus flare-ups emphasizes how critical it is to address the mind-body link.

Stress reduction and relaxation are greatly enhanced by mindfulness-based activities like yoga and meditation. These activities provide a more balanced physiological environment in addition to improving mental health.

Furthermore, the effectiveness of cognitive-behavioral therapy (CBT) in assisting people in managing chronic conditions, such as lupus, has come to light. Through the examination of thinking processes and actions, cognitive behavioral therapy (CBT) gives people useful skills for stress management and mental resilience building. Understanding how the mind affects lupus symptoms is a crucial part of a lupus diet because it encourages people to think about their overall health in terms of not just nutrition but also emotional and psychological aspects.

Long-Term Plans for the Wellness of Lupus:

The path of managing lupus demands the adoption of long-term, sustainable methods for total wellness in addition to urgent symptom treatment.

Maintaining a nutrient-rich, well-balanced diet that boosts immunity and reduces inflammation is one such tactic. A diet low in processed foods and possible triggers and high in complete foods—such as fruits, vegetables, lean meats, and omega-3 fatty acids—is recommended for people with lupus.

A further essential component of long-term lupus wellness is regular physical activity. Exercise that is customized for each person's skills helps to enhance cardiovascular health, muscle strength, and general energy. However, it's important for people with lupus to exercise according to their unique needs and to work with medical professionals to create a safe and efficient fitness program.

Long-term lupus management also rests on regular medical monitoring and discussion with healthcare specialists. Frequent examinations, blood marker monitoring, and honest discussion about symptoms enable patients and their medical team to make well-informed decisions and modify the treatment plan as necessary.

Essentially, developing a lupus-friendly lifestyle is about committing to long-term health by combining physical, dietary, and medical approaches.

~ 87 ~

www.ingramcontent.com/pod-product-compliance
Lightning Source LLC
Chambersburg PA
CBHW060754260726
48660CB00002B/619